WELCOME TO THE CELEBRITY SLIM PROGRAMME

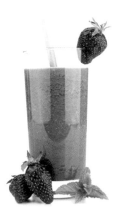

The Celebrity Slim Programme is a simple and effective weight loss programme* designed to help you lose weight and to keep it off for good. There are no gimmicks and no calorie counting, it's just an easy to follow programme which helps you achieve some great results!

Simply replace 2 meals each day from a huge variety of delicious Celebrity Slim shakes, soups and bars, eat one healthy balanced meal, and snack up to three times on a range of tasty foods. It's that easy!

This guide will take you through the dos and don'ts of the programme

• What you can eat and drink

• Food and drinks that should be avoided

• How you can expect to feel

• How your body will adjust to your new way of eating

The Celebrity Slim Programme is designed to help you reach your target weight. Once you're there, we'll show you how to eat to maintain your new shape and stay feeling your best.

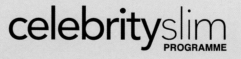

*Healthy and effective weight loss when substituting two daily meals with meal replacement products from the Celebrity Slim energy restricted diet and exercise programme.

Welcome

THERE ARE THREE PHASES TO CHOOSE FROM IN THE CELEBRITY SLIM PROGRAMME EACH OF WHICH HAS BEEN DESIGNED TO ACHIEVE A SPECIFIC GOAL.

The Celebrity Slim Phases

If you are new to Celebrity Slim you can start on any of the three phases depending on your goal.

THE TRIM PHASE
long-term sustainable results

The TRIM Phase is at the heart of the programme and is designed to deliver long-term sustainable results. This is the classic phase where you replace 2 meals each day and combine this with a balanced meal and up to 3 snacks. This easy-to-follow programme allows you to eat regularly and is flexible enough to fit in with your work and home life. This guide contains all of the information and guidance you need to make the TRIM Phase work for you.

> **2 Celebrity Slim meal replacements**
> **3 snacks • 1 balanced meal • 2L water**

THE ACTIVE PHASE
kick-start your diet

The ACTIVE Phase can get your diet off to a great start or help if your weight loss has plateaued. This short phase combines 3 ACTIVE Shakes each day with a balanced meal and, most importantly, 20-30 minutes moderate daily exercise. Find out more about the ACTIVE Phase later in this guide.

> **3 Celebrity Slim Active Shakes • 1 balanced meal**
> **•2L water • 20-30 min moderate daily exercise**

THE MAINTAIN PHASE
keep it off for good

The MAINTAIN Phase is designed to help you keep the weight off for good once you have reached you target weight. The Celebrity Slim Programme is about changing your eating habits so that you lose weight and, importantly, stay feeling your best. This phase helps you firmly establish your new healthy eating habits. We have included a section later in this guide to steer you through this stage and help you keep making the right food choices.

> 1 Celebrity Slim meal replacement • 3 snacks
> 2 balanced meals (with moderate carbohydrate) • 2L water

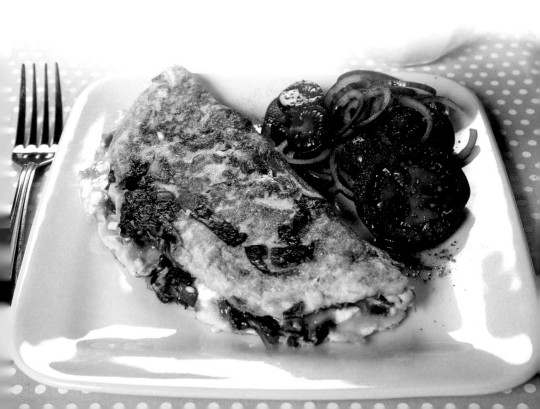

TRIM PHASE
TO REACH YOUR GOAL

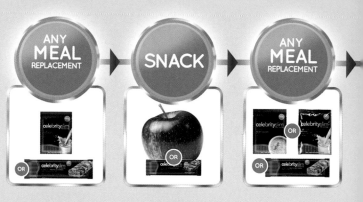

ANY MEAL REPLACEMENT → **SNACK** → **ANY MEAL REPLACEMENT** →

• Use ANY meal replacement from the range • Eat 6 times a day

ACTIVE PHASE
TO KICK START YOUR DIET

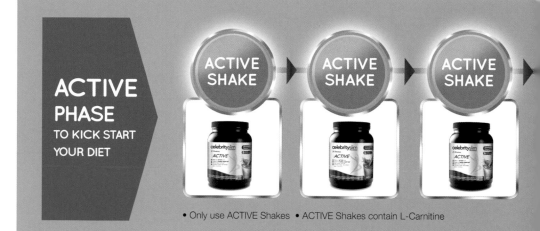

ACTIVE SHAKE → **ACTIVE SHAKE** → **ACTIVE SHAKE** →

• Only use ACTIVE Shakes • ACTIVE Shakes contain L-Carnitine

MAINTAIN PHASE
TO KEEP IT OFF

ANY MEAL REPLACEMENT → **SNACK** → **BALANCED MEAL** →

• Use any meal replacement from the range at either breakfast, lunch or dinner

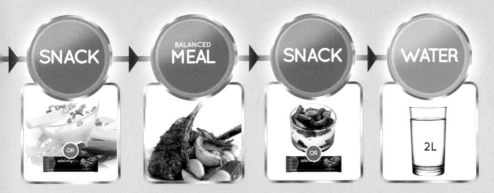

• Exercise is recommended but not compulsory • Alcohol should only be consumed in moderation

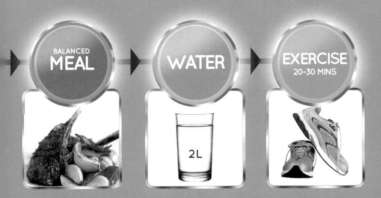

• A minimum of 20 - 30 minutes moderate daily exercise must be incorporated • No snacks or alcohol allowed

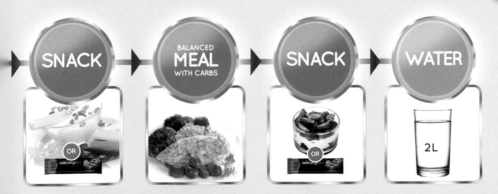

• Exercise is recommended but not compulsory • Alcohol should only be consumed in moderation

The Phases

HOW DOES THE CELEBRITY SLIM PROGRAMME WORK?

The Celebrity Slim Programme is a nutritionally balanced diet plan, proven to help you lose weight and maintain your new figure.*

Put simply, the Celebrity Slim Programme works by reducing the amount of overall carbohydrates and calories in your diet, creating an energy deficiency, which leads to weight loss.
Our products are packed full of 3 sources of protein, along with 25 Essential Vitamins and Minerals to support your metabolism and help you get the nutrients your body needs.

Eating regularly can help reduce hunger cravings so on the Celebrity Slim Programme we ask you to **eat 6 times a day,** combining regular snacks and a balanced meal with your Celebrity Slim Meal replacements.

Cutting back on carbohydrates

The carbohydrates you eat, such as sugar, bread, pasta and rice are your body's primary source of energy. Carbohydrates are stored in your body as sugars in your muscles and liver; excess carbohydrates that are not used by your body are stored as fat.

When you start changing the way you eat your body continues to burn carbohydrates for energy. If you cut back on the amount of carbohydrates you eat your stores will run low, which forces your body to start burning more fat for energy, so you lose weight faster.

In a typical western diet we tend to eat far more carbohydrates than we need, so the Celebrity Slim Programme aims to reduce the amount of carbohydrates in your diet. It is not a "no" or "low" carbohydrate diet but a moderate carbohydrate programme. You will still consume approximately 100g of carbohydrates per day.

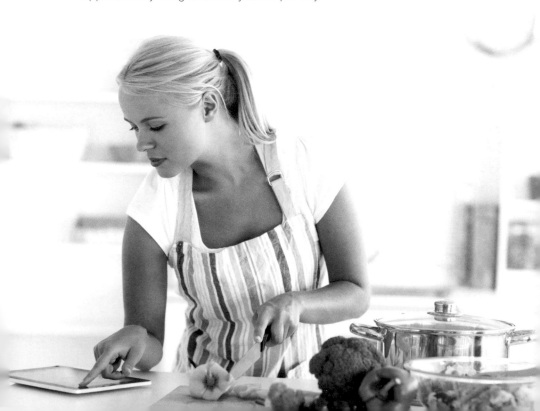

What about Calories?

It's important to have a basic understanding of how much energy is in the food you eat. The energy value of food is measured in Calories **(kcal)** and sometimes in kilojoules **(kj)**. Many diets focus on counting Calories, but with Celebrity Slim you don't need to. Simply by following Celebrity Slim you'll not only cut back the amount of carbohydrates you eat but you will almost certainly reduce your overall Calorie intake as well. That's because our guidelines will help you make healthier, low-Calorie, food choices and the Calorie content of our meal replacements is carefully controlled.

Almost everyone has a different daily energy requirement, which is determined by many factors such as age, sex, body type, health status and level of physical activity. The daily amount of Calories your body requires to function is looked at on two levels:

1. Basal Metabolic Rate (BMR) – this is the amount of energy your body uses to function when at rest or sleeping.

2. Active Metabolic Rate – the extra energy you burn through your activity during the day such as walking, working, housework, etc.

FEWER CALORIES IN   **MORE** CALORIES OUT

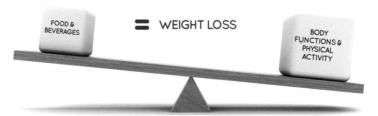

FOOD & BEVERAGES   **= WEIGHT LOSS**   BODY FUNCTIONS & PHYSICAL ACTIVITY

With Celebrity Slim you will control your overall Calorie intake to below your body's required level, using your internal fat stores for energy, which should result in weight loss.

Eating smaller meals more often

Reducing Calories is important but it is not the whole story. Eating smaller meals, more regularly, is also a key element of the Celebrity Slim Programme. Many dieters spend much of their day eating very little, but then eat 1 or 2 larger meals with the belief that starving for most of the day will help them lose weight.

In fact, the opposite is true.

When you 'starve' yourself for maybe 5–6 hours, a number of physiological changes occur in your body. After around 3 hours without eating, your blood sugars begin to drop and will cause you to feel quite hungry. If you have a meal at this point, your hunger means you're at risk of overeating. You may also find you crave something sweet or starchy – that's your body's way of looking for carbohydrates as a quick fix to restore its blood sugar balance.

 If you don't eat anything and continue to fast, your metabolism starts to lapse into what's called 'starvation mode'. Your hunger pains may go away, but this is a sign your metabolism is starting to slow down as your body starts to conserve energy. This is the opposite of what you want, as when your body conserves energy, fat burning slows down, making weight loss more difficult.

We can avoid this phenomenon with the simple trick of eating every few hours, which means about 5–6 meals spaced out during each day and by keeping fully hydrated. By eating and drinking regularly, your blood sugars remain stable, you don't get overly hungry, and you are less likely to overeat at each meal.

The Importance of Protein

Protein is a key ingredient in our meal replacement products and we ask you to eat a good source of protein at every main meal occasion. **There are two key benefits** to increasing the amount of protein in your diet alongside a reduction in carbohydrates.

Firstly, whilst researchers are not sure of the exact cause, this combination appears to help reduce appetite and cravings so that you are not constantly hungry.

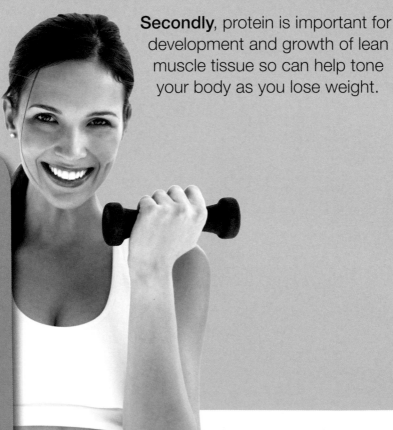

Secondly, protein is important for development and growth of lean muscle tissue so can help tone your body as you lose weight.

How it works

Positive Habits

Many traditional diets feel like a punishment where you are denied your favourite foods until the weight is lost. Once you reach your goal and are free of the restriction, you can't wait to go back to your old ways and this is the reason so many people struggle to maintain their weight loss.

From our experience the secret is to make the programme feel like a positive, sustainable experience that fits in with your lifestyle. If you are losing weight and feeling great there is no reason why you should be overweight again. Being able to eat regularly, to enjoy a variety of great-tasting products and to discover simple, new ways of enhancing your meals, all helps to make your weight loss journey a more positive experience. At Celebrity Slim we are determined to give you the tools to make long term weight management a reality.

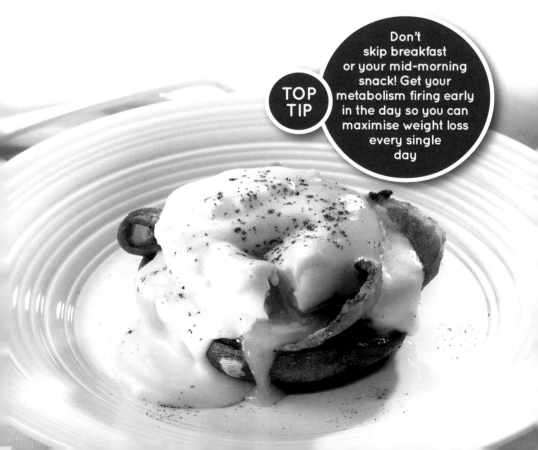

TOP TIP

Don't skip breakfast or your mid-morning snack! Get your metabolism firing early in the day so you can maximise weight loss every single day

KEYS TO WEIGHT LOSS SUCCESS

✓ **Calorie Reduction**
You will consume between 1200-1500 Calories per day.

✓ **Controlling Carbohydrates**
Your daily carbohydrate intake will fall from an average of 250-350g to 90-150g.

✓ **Choose Good Fats**
Whilst overall fat consumption will be reduced you will still consume sufficient essential 'good fats'.

✓ **Protein at each meal**
This helps to provide adequate protein for lean muscle maintenance.

✓ **Better food choices**
We help you to make better choices: low GI carbohydrates and healthy fats.

✓ **Plenty of fruit and vegetables**
We recommend you consume 2 low GI fruits and 3 servings of vegetables per day to help increase your vitamin, mineral, anti-oxidant and fibre intake.

✓ **Smaller portion size**
Smaller and more regular portion sizes mean we do not over-consume in one meal and we spread our intake throughout the day.

✓ **Water consumption**
Water plays a key part in the Celebrity Slim Programme. You should aim to drink 2 litres of water each day.

✓ **Support**
Support is available every step of the way through our trained staff, our website or our call centre.

Celebrity Slim Meal Replacements

The Celebrity Slim Programme combines Celebrity Slim products with a healthy eating plan. Central to the programme are the Celebrity Slim Meal Replacement products which should replace 2 of your daily meals on the TRIM Phase.

These products are designed to give you all of the nutrients you need to keep your body functioning healthily but have also been carefully developed to keep carbohydrates low and proteins high.

That way your food intake at these 2 meals each day is closely controlled. In addition we recognise that variety and flavour are important factors in helping you stick to a diet programme, so we have developed great-tasting products for you to enjoy.

For many of our customers **Celebrity Slim Shakes** are at the heart of the diet. Our easy-to-use shakes are formulated to be made with water making them handy for use both at home and at work. They are best made using the **Celebrity Slim Shaker** which will give the shake a light and frothy texture.

The shakes are available in a wide range of flavours from favourites such as chocolate and strawberry to café latte and vanilla. If you are out and about, look out for our ready-to-drink shakes which are perfect to pop into your bag for lunch.

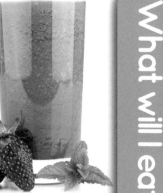

Check out the range at: **celebrityslim.co.uk**

What will I eat?

If you feel you want a change from shakes try one of our range of **Celebrity Slim Meal Replacement Bars** such as the moreish Fruit and Nut Bar. These bars are designed to satisfy your sweet tooth and your hunger in one go. One bar provides all the nutrients you need from a meal.

For a savoury option we have a range of **Celebrity Slim Soups** - a perfect, comforting lunchtime option for cooler months.

Our popular soups allow you to keep your diet varied and interesting. Choose from old favourites Roast Chicken and Garden Vegetable or the more exotic Mild Curry.

Sign up online and receive regular updates on new products.

what will I eat?

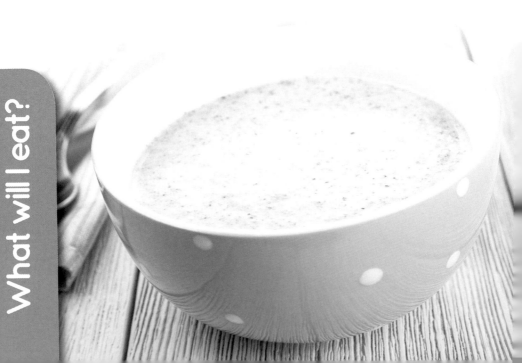

Balanced Meal

Each day you'll eat one balanced meal - most popularly lunch or dinner – which should consist of a good quality protein source such as meat, fish or poultry, accompanied by a healthy selection of salad or vegetables.

For vegetarian options try eggs, Quorn™ or low-fat cheeses such as ricotta. It's amazing how many delicious, satisfying meals can be created from this simple meal formula. To help you plan we have pulled together some great, simple recipes and ideas for meals in this Guide and you can find many more on our website.

 The main point to remember when planning your balanced meal is to avoid carbohydrate rich foods such as bread, rice, pasta and potatoes as including these foods in your meals will affect your weight-loss results.

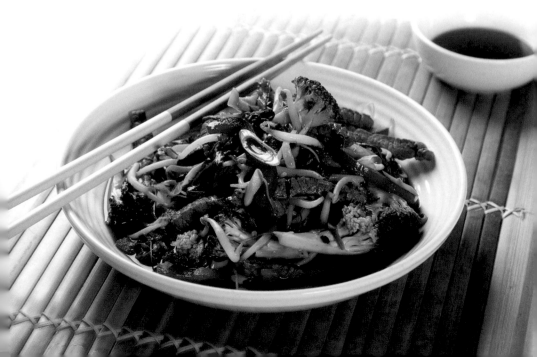

Protein Foods

Most protein foods generally contain some fats, so you should be looking for lean meat with little fat and where there is fat do your best to ensure that all excess fat is removed prior to cooking or serving. This is a great rule for longer term healthy eating as much of the fat on meat and poultry is saturated fat which can lead to increased cholesterol levels in the blood and a number of associated health risks.

The recommended portion size of protein should be between 100g–150g (uncooked weight) for women and 100g–200g (uncooked weight) for men. As a general rule, the portion should be about the size and thickness of the palm of your hand.

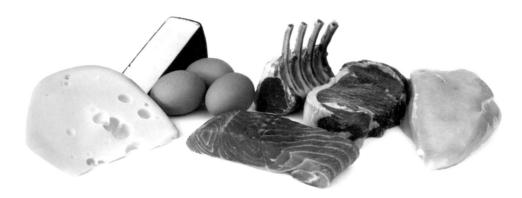

Recognising Carbohydrates

It can be difficult to recognise carbohydrate-rich foods, particularly when they are fresh foods and may not be clearly labelled.

For example, some fruits and vegetables contain more sugars and starch than others and therefore have a higher carbohydrate level.

These higher carb vegetables and fruits should be avoided on the Celebrity Slim Programme. To help you find your way easily to the best food options we have also created a handy list of foods to enjoy and foods to avoid. You can find all of this information at the back of this guide.

Vegetables

A variety of vegetables will help keep your meals healthy. Colourful and tasty, vegetables are not only delicious but packed full of essential nutrients such as vitamins and minerals. You should aim to eat at least 3 good servings of vegetables each day from the list on page 69, whilst avoiding the high carbohydrate vegetables. As a general guide, your dinner plate should consist of approximately one third protein and two thirds vegetables.

There are some vegetables you'll need to avoid – typically these are the starchy ones like potato, parsnip and sweetcorn. The lists at the back of this guide separates the two to make it easier for you to make the right choices.

Adding Flavour

Herbs and spices, sauces and condiments transform simple ingredients into delicious meals and the more flavour you can pack into your dishes the more satisfied you will feel. Try using simple, natural ingredients such as olive oil, soy sauce, lemon juice, balsamic or normal vinegar, and tomato puree. Garlic and fresh herbs such as basil, parsley, chives, mint or coriander will freshen up chicken and fish or try more exotic dried herbs and spices such as chilli, curry powder, oregano, paprika, cumin, or ginger. Worcestershire sauce is a great condiment for adding spice and depth of flavour to dishes. When using ready made sauces or dressings remember to choose low carbohydrate or diet options.

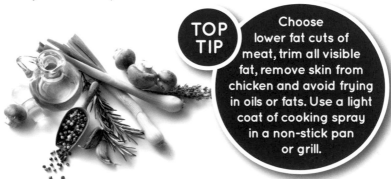

TOP TIP Choose lower fat cuts of meat, trim all visible fat, remove skin from chicken and avoid frying in oils or fats. Use a light coat of cooking spray in a non-stick pan or grill.

We have put together some simple meal ideas that will help to take the stress out of your planning, whilst delivering delicious meals to your table. Don't forget what is healthy for you is also healthy for your family and friends, so you can serve the same recipes to others with rice, pasta or potatoes, simply avoid the carbohydrate yourself. Check out some more of our recipes at the back of this guide they are just a small selection from a range of recipes that we have had developed to make planning your meals easier. Many more appetising recipes that cater for a wide range of tastes are available on our website and our downloadable APP - for FREE!

Some simple examples of a balanced meal

- Grilled marinated chicken breast with a tossed salad of lettuce, spring onions, tomatoes, mangetout and avocado with Low-Calorie Italian dressing.

- Steak and mushrooms with steamed broccoli, courgette, green beans and carrots.

- Lamb curry served with steamed spinach.

- Stir fried chicken and vegetables including broccoli, pak choi, red pepper, water chestnuts and bean shoots.

- Spanish omelette (2 eggs, cheese, diced tomato, diced onion) with bacon and salad.

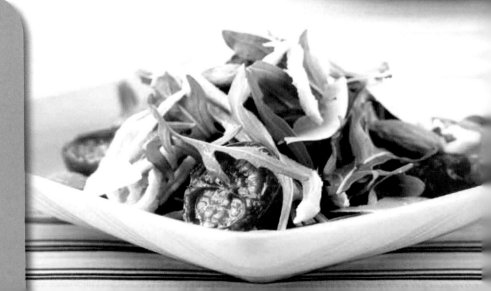

What will I eat?

Snack Foods

The Celebrity Slim eating guidelines allow you to have 3 snacks each day to help keep those hunger cravings at bay and provide variety and interest to your diet.

Many people choose to eat fruit for their snacks during the day, or fruit with yoghurt in the evening, but if you fancy a savoury snack there are lots of options to choose from such as vegetables, nuts or cheese. One of the great things about Celebrity Slim is that it is flexible and allows you to choose what you eat, just remember to follow the core programme guidelines, watch portion sizes and avoid carbohydrate rich, high fat and sugary foods.

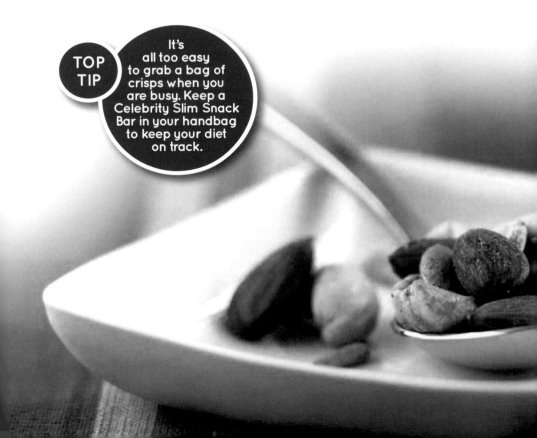

TOP TIP

It's all too easy to grab a bag of crisps when you are busy. Keep a Celebrity Slim Snack Bar in your handbag to keep your diet on track.

Below are some suitable snack foods and ideas that are relatively low in both Calories and carbohydrates, and won't upset the programme. In addition there is a range of **Celebrity Slim Snack Bars** available if you want a satisfying sweet snack, such as the indulgent Sticky Toffee bars or satisfying Rocky Road bars. If you are unsure or want more snack ideas turn to the back of this guide, visit our website or call the Celebrity Slim helpline.

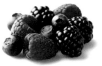

1/2 to 3/4 cup fresh or frozen berries

Small apple or orange, medium peach or plum

Small block of cheese (30g) or 1 to 2 slices of lean deli meat such as ham

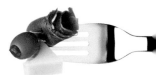

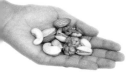

A small handful (30g) of nuts such as raw almonds, peanuts, Brazil nuts or pistachios (go easy on salted nuts and avoid any coated nuts).

Carrot and/or celery sticks with cream cheese or low fat dip

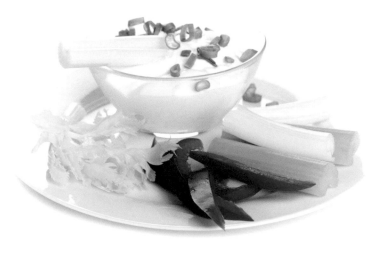

What will I eat?

DRINKS

Water accounts for around 60% of the body weight of the average adult so the amount of water we consume can make a huge difference to how we feel both physically and mentally. Dehydration often leads to headaches, tiredness and mood swings, which can make it harder to stick to a new diet programme.

As a key part of the Celebrity Slim Programme we ask you to drink around 2L, or 8 glasses of water each day. This may seem a lot but it is in line with healthy guidelines and will help to make you feel more alert, support your digestion and keep you feeling full. More importantly it establishes water consumption as a healthy habit, so that even when you reach your weight loss goals you continue to reap the health benefits of water consumption.

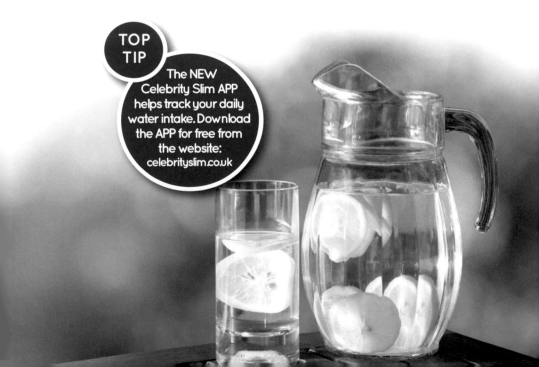

TOP TIP

The NEW Celebrity Slim APP helps track your daily water intake. Download the APP for free from the website: celebrityslim.co.uk

Combine your daily water intake with other drinks such as tea and coffee (a maximum of 3 cups of tea or coffee can be consumed per day) and diet soft drinks, in moderation, throughout the day.
Fruit and herb teas are a great choice as they are Calorie free and come in a range of flavours.

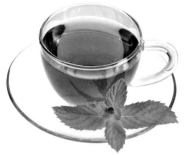

 Other fruit-based drinks such as pure fruit juices, fruit smoothies and full sugar soft drinks are high in sugar and should be avoided.

While there is nothing wrong with having an occasional alcoholic drink, drinking too much can be harmful to your health. Research shows that drinking too much alcohol increases your chances of having high blood pressure and heavy drinking can also lead to a wide range of health problems. Keeping your alcohol consumption at a sensible level will help you develop positive habits for the future.

In addition to the associated health risks, alcohol often has a high Calorie content and we recommend you reduce your consumption to maximise weight loss and improve overall health.

Within the Celebrity Slim Programme guidelines you can still treat yourself to a glass of wine or a small, low-carbohydrate beer, 2-3 days per week. Use a smaller glass (125ml) and choose a dry white or red wine rather than a sweet white or rose, as these contain more sugar and therefore more Calories. Similarly if you prefer to drink a spirit, ensure that it is a single measure and try to mix with a diet mixer such as slimline tonic, soda water, diet coke or diet lemonade. Check out the full drink guidelines at the back of this guide.

GETTING STARTED
SETTING YOUR
WEIGHT LOSS GOAL.

Most big achievements in life are a direct result of having set a clear goal, and striving towards it. Weight loss is no different. Your goal may not be just to do with weight - it could be one of the following;

- Fitting into your favourite clothes
- Dropping a dress size
- Having more energy
- Feeling better about yourself
- Improving your health and wellbeing
- Preparing for a holiday or wedding

TOP TIP

To automatically calculate your BMI, go to our website and enter your information into our BMI Calculator.

Whatever your goal is take a moment to imagine yourself weeks or months into the future when you have made it! Imagine the sense of achievement and confidence you will get from having taken the important step to lose weight and from sticking with it.

Your goal weight

Setting a realistic target weight is an important part of the Celebrity Slim Programme. Goals need to be both short and long term, so before you get started make sure you know what you're aiming for.

WHAT IS A REALISTIC TARGET WEIGHT TO SET?

We understand that people have different reasons for losing weight and your weight loss target will vary depending upon your starting weight and your reasons for wanting to lose weight. The key to success is to be realistic and set achievable goals. Remember, you can always set new goals once you've reached your initial target.

We would recommend targeting no more than **10%** weight loss from your starting weight. A **10%** drop can have a massive impact on the way you feel and your general health. Once you have reached your target, and if you still have weight to lose, you can set yourself a new target to aim for.

The best way to achieve a goal is to make **small changes** along the way. The Celebrity Slim Programme will help you do this through the simple and structured plan that educates you on healthy habits for life. A practical tool to help keep you motivated towards your weight loss goal is to track your progress.

We recommend you weigh yourself and maybe take measurements of your waist or hips, or take a few 'before' photos. After each week weigh and measure yourself and record your progress. Use our handy diary pages at the back of this guide, or the Celebrity Slim APP, to track your progress.

Why not break your goal down into weekly chunks and have a list of rewards for when each week's goal is attained, something small to make you feel good about yourself and inspire you to keep achieving. Don't worry if you have a bad week - this can sometimes simply be the result of your body's natural cycle.

Getting Started

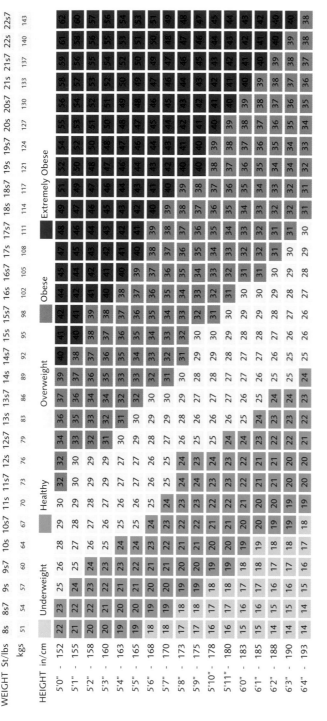

Body Mass Index (BMI)

The medically preferred method of determining a healthy weight is called the Body Mass Index or BMI. Your BMI is a number calculated from your weight and height. Use the table above to find your current BMI and weight classification. In general Celebrity Slim is suitable for people in the overweight category or above but you may be at the higher end of the healthy category and only have a small amount of weight you want to lose, or you may wish to follow the MAINTAIN Phase to help keep your weight at a healthy level. It is important that people with a BMI of over 30 consult their GP before embarking on any diet programme.

TOP TIP

Weigh yourself at the same time each week and in similar clothes. First thing in the morning is best. Watching your weight steadily reduce is very motivating!

THE TRIM PHASE
IS DESIGNED
TO ACHIEVE
LONG-TERM
SUSTAINABLE
RESULTS

THE TRIM PHASE

Before starting, it's important to consider your timing. Is there any reason you may find it more difficult to stick to the eating plans? Don't try to start if you are about to go away on holidays, or if you know you will be in an environment where meal planning will be difficult. Try and give yourself the best chance of succeeding right from the beginning; settle on a starting point and get going!

The aim of the first week is to reduce the amount of carbohydrates you eat and increase the amount of protein. This in turn will change your body from using mainly carbohydrates as fuel to using more fats. It is extremely important to follow the programme strictly and not eat any carbohydrate rich foods during this week or the programme simply will not work.

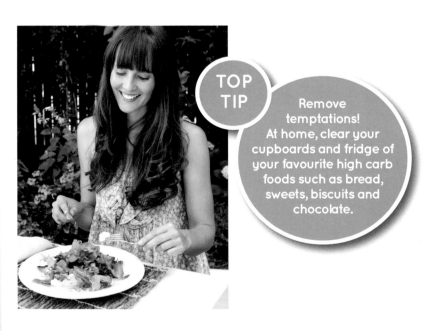

TOP TIP

Remove temptations! At home, clear your cupboards and fridge of your favourite high carb foods such as bread, sweets, biscuits and chocolate.

CHECKLIST- THE TRIM PHASE

✓ **DO** replace 2 meals each day with Celebrity Slim Meal Replacement products

✓ **DO** plan your balanced meal each day
- planning your food helps you to keep on track.

✓ **DO** remember to drink 2 litres of water each day

✓ **DO** have your 3 allowable snacks each day

✓ **DO** eat the correct types of fruit & vegetables

✓ **DO** keep referring to your Programme Guide

✓ **DO** join the Celebrity Slim Club for FREE
- at www.celebrityslim.co.uk

✓ **DO** start to think about exercise
- turn to page 46 for some ideas.

✗ **Don't** forget to say "no" to the following foods
- potatoes, rice, pasta, bread, bananas, grapes.

✗ **Don't** weigh yourself every day
Your weight can fluctuate day to day, keep to once a week.

✗ **Don't** give up!
Losing weight isn't easy but the results will be worth it.

AN EXAMPLE OF A TYPICAL WEEK ON

	Day 1	Day 2	Day 3
Breakfast **Meal**	Celebrity Slim Strawberry Shake	Celebrity Slim Cafe Latte Shake	Celebrity Slim Fruit & Nut Meal Bar
Mid Morning **Snack**	Crunchy apple	Chunk of cheese	Celebrity Slim Rocky Road Snack Bar
Lunch **Meal**	Celebrity Slim Chicken Soup	Celebrity Slim Choc Meal Bar	Celebrity Slim Chocolate Shak
Mid Afternoon **Snack**	Small handful of nuts	Crunchy apple	Hummus with crudités
Dinner **Balanced Meal**	Grilled chicken with wholegrain mustard, green beans & broccoli	Oriental salmon & mixed stir fry vegetables	Steak with celer mash and spina
Supper **Snack**	Small orange	Celebrity Slim Sticky Toffee Snack Bar	Crunchy appl

The first week of any new programme can be hard as your body adjusts to a new way of eating. Bear with it and after a week you should start to feel more energetic and healthier than you have for some time. There are a few tell tale signs that the Celebrity Slim Programme is working:

- After a few days you may get cravings for sweet foods - resist these by eating your allowable snacks! This is a good sign that your carbohydrates are running low and that your body is starting to burn more fat.

- After about a week to 10 days you will be surprised to find your cravings and hunger reduce dramatically and it's far easier to stay on the programme – most people find they have more energy and feel great!

The Trim Phase

THE TRIM PHASE

Day 4	Day 5	Day 6	Day 7
Celebrity Slim Cafe Latte Shake	Celebrity Slim Vanilla Shake	Celebrity Slim Strawberry Shake	Celebrity Slim Fruit & Nut Meal Bar
Celebrity Slim Sticky Toffee Snack Bar	2 Slices of lean ham	Celebrity Slim Rocky Road Snack Bar	Grilled mushrooms topped with grated cheese
Celebrity Slim Garden Vegetable Soup	Celebrity Slim Fruit & Nut Bar	Celebrity Slim Meal Bar	Celebrity Slim Vanilla Shake
Small orange	Crunchy apple	Crudités with low fat dip	Celebrity Slim Cranberry Yogurt Snack bar
Frittata with chorizo, spinach & ricotta, grilled tomatoes & mushrooms	Tuna with tomatoes, garlic & olives & courgettes	Chicken breast with ricotta & prosciutto, rocket salad with parmesan	Roast beef with leeks, cauliflower & carrots
Chunk of cheese with celery sticks	Low fat raspberry yogurt	Mixed berries with low fat natural yogurt	Celery sticks and low fat cream cheese

- Because you're drinking more water and your body is flushing out toxins that are naturally produced from breaking down fat, you may need to visit the loo more often - this is a good sign. It is important to remember to drink at least 2 litres of water a day to assist with flushing out these toxins.

- As your body adjusts to the programme and the changes in your eating habits, you may experience a dull headache or feel lethargic for a day or two – don't be concerned, this will pass. Make sure you are drinking the recommended 2 litres of water each day, as this will help to ease any headaches.

STAYING THE COURSE

After your first week your body and mind should be getting used to Celebrity Slim Meal Replacements and your lower carbohydrate, higher protein meals.

You don't really need to change anything from your first week to continue to manage your weight. Simply stick with your 2 Celebrity Slim Meal Replacements (shakes, soups, smoothie, ready meals or bars), one balanced meal and your allowable snacks each day. However, if you're planning to stay on the programme for several weeks or months, it is worthwhile exploring a variety of different recipes to keep your balanced meal choices interesting and something to look forward to. Don't forget our great range of recipe ideas for the Celebrity Slim Programme on the website and the APP.

Eating out

When you prepare and eat your meals at home, it's relatively easy to keep to your eating plan. However, dining away from home, whether it's a quick takeaway or the finest 5 star restaurant, offers some challenges, but sensible planning and choosing when you're out will help you keep within the programme guidelines.

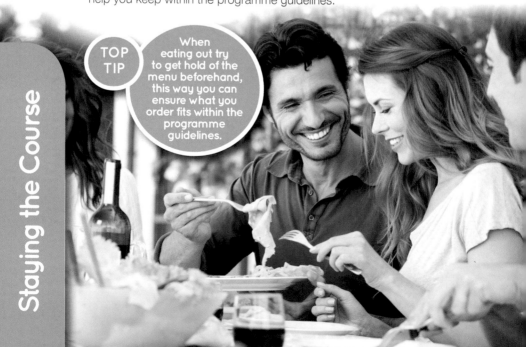

TOP TIP

When eating out try to get hold of the menu beforehand, this way you can ensure what you order fits within the programme guidelines.

Take away food

Almost all fast food, pizza, fish and chips, burgers and pies, are high in carbohydrates and should be avoided. If you find yourself looking for a fast food option **here are a few take away suggestions to consider**:

- Many Asian dishes, such as stir fries, offer a more healthy option. Just remember not to eat the rice or noodles and avoid dishes with sweet sauces such as sweet and sour, lemon chicken or sweet chilli, as these will be high in sugar.
- Chicken and beef satay sticks with satay sauce are delicious and contain very few carbohydrates.
- Takeaway chicken, beef or tuna salads tend to be low in carbohydrates provided they aren't pasta salads.
- If you love Indian food look for sauce-free dishes such as chicken tandoori, and avoid cream-based sauces, opting instead for sauces based on tomato.

Remember to think about portion size - fast food portions can be much bigger than we would recommend. Be sensible about the food you choose - look at the menu and go for the low carbohydrate alternatives. A salad instead of a sandwich, a chicken kebab instead of a chicken korma.

Restaurant dining

- Ask the waiter to explain what vegetables are served with any main course
- Replace potatoes, rice and pasta with low carb vegetables or salad.

- Avoid temptations such as bread rolls, garlic bread, etc.
- It's always better to choose a starter and main course rather than a main course and dessert which is more likely to be higher in carbohydrates and fats.
- Make your wine last longer by combining with sparkling water as a spritzer or simply ensuring that you take 2 sips of water to every sip of wine as you eat.

Eating at work

If you need to eat meals at work, then simply take a shake, soup, smoothie or bar for your lunch and make sure you are prepared for your mid-morning and afternoon snacks. That way you can avoid feeling hungry and being tempted by the office biscuit supply. At the start of each working week, **write down your snack times, plan what you'll eat** and then stock up on the foods you need. After a few weeks this will become second nature.

Living & Eating with Others

If you're living on your own, it's relatively easy to adjust your lifestyle to suit the Celebrity Slim Programme. If you live with others you will most likely be confronted with more temptation in the kitchen, as your housemates or family members continue to eat high carbohydrate foods. Explain the programme to the others - you'll usually find everyone is supportive.

Remember, you can enjoy a balanced meal each day, which means you can continue to share meals with family or friends
– simply avoiding any carbohydrate which is served alongside and making sure you eat plenty of extra vegetables or salad. Ultimately your family or friends will also benefit from the healthier foods you serve.

Thinking about exercise

Whilst the Celebrity Slim TRIM Phase is designed to be effective whether or not you exercise, why not think about introducing some exercise into your daily routine as it will help to burn fat faster.
Take a look at the section on page 46 for some ideas and inspiration.

WHAT TO DO IF YOU SLIP UP

Let's face it, it's almost impossible to stay on any diet or eating plan for an extended period and not slip up sometimes. It's normal, and it's not the end of the world. But if you're serious about reaching your goal weight, it's what you do after you slip up that's important. The sooner you get back on to the Celebrity Slim Programme, the sooner you'll go back to controlling your weight.

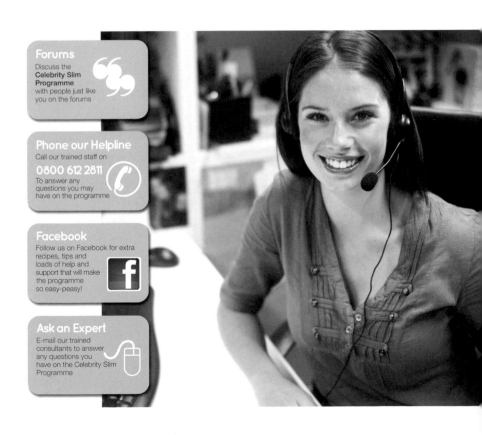

Forums
Discuss the **Celebrity Slim Programme** with people just like you on the forums

Phone our Helpline
Call our trained staff on
0800 612 2811
To answer any questions you may have on the programme

Facebook
Follow us on Facebook for extra recipes, tips and loads of help and support that will make the programme so easy-peasy!

Ask an Expert
E-mail our trained consultants to answer any questions you have on the Celebrity Slim Programme

IF YOU NEED SUPPORT

Sticking to a weight-loss programme is not easy – you will most probably have good days when you feel confident and sure of your decisions and others where you feel like giving up. Life goes on whilst you are trying to diet and other issues at home, at work, with friends or with family, can affect the choices you make each day. At the same time, as you start to introduce new foods into your diet you may have questions regarding whether they fit within the programme.

We understand that you may need advice and support at any time throughout your diet so we have made sure this is available for you when, and where, you want it. Whether you want advice on what to eat, are struggling with temptation or have come to a difficult point in your weight loss, there are ways to get all the answers you need. Call the Celebrity Slim helpline to speak to a trained advisor who can give you personalised advice on any aspect of the programme. If you prefer to email, that option is also available to you on the Ask an Expert section of the website.

KEEP IN TOUCH

Sometimes it can help to speak to someone in the same situation as you, so you may want to check out our active social forums on the website and on Facebook, where you can get advice and support from fellow dieters. It makes sense to sign-up to the **Celebrity Slim Club online** to keep abreast of news, recipes and ideas to help you towards your goals, along with bespoke offers and great prize draw promotions. **Membership is completely FREE** and members have access to a wealth of recipes and can also browse the full product range. Signing up is quick and easy – simply go to **celebrityslim.co.uk** and on **Facebook** (https://www.facebook.com/celebrityslimukandireland) to find out more.

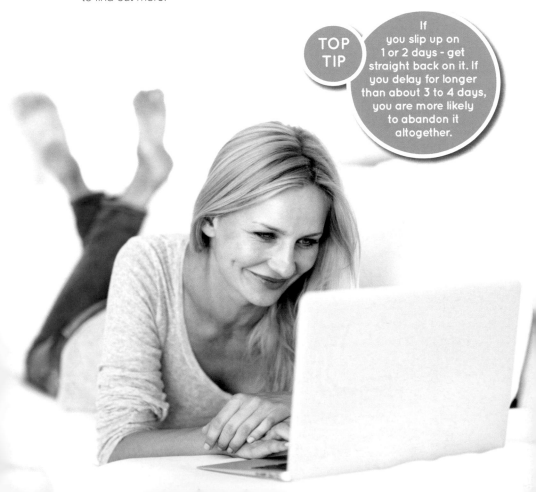

TOP TIP

If you slip up on 1 or 2 days - get straight back on it. If you delay for longer than about 3 to 4 days, you are more likely to abandon it altogether.

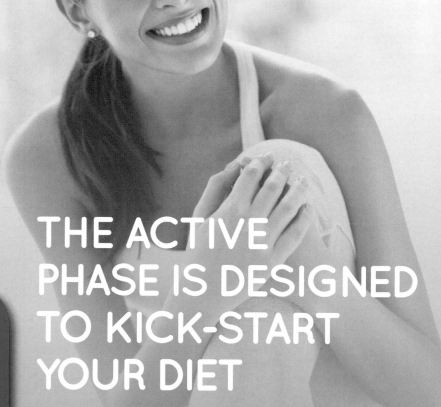

THE ACTIVE PHASE IS DESIGNED TO KICK-START YOUR DIET

THE ACTIVE PHASE

If you enjoy exercise then you may be interested in our ACTIVE Phase, which combines exercise with Celebrity Slim ACTIVE Shakes to get your diet off to a great start. You simply consume 3 ACTIVE Shakes, spaced through the day, along with a balanced meal and importantly, 2 litres of water.

The Celebrity Slim ACTIVE Phase has been devised to closely control your overall daily Calorie and carbohydrate intake without the need for complicated Calorie counting. It is simple and easy to follow and when combined with exercise encourages the body to burn fat leading to weight loss.* It's a great option if you want to kick-start your diet or when you feel your weight loss has started to plateau and you need a boost.

In the ACTIVE Phase you must commit to exercise each day, which will not only burn extra calories, but can also begin to establish exercise as part of your healthy lifestyle. You should aim for 20-30 minutes of moderate exercise each day, remembering to start at a manageable level and build up from there. Walking, swimming, cycling or even vigorous housework can all count as exercise. The main thing is to get ACTIVE!

*Studies show that substituting two daily meals with meal replacements helps to lose weight in the context of an energy restricted diet and exercise programme.

CHECKLIST - THE ACTIVE PHASE

✓ **DO** drink at least 2 litres of water each day
This is especially important since you are exercising

✓ **DO** make sure you exercise each day
- for 20-30 minutes

✓ **DO** find an exercise-buddy
Exercising with a friend or in a group can be more fun!

✓ **DO** have plenty of vegetables or salad
- with your balanced meal as this will help add fibre to your diet

✓ **DO** refer to the Programme Guide Eating Guidelines

✗ **Don't** drink alcohol
It is not allowed on the ACTIVE Phase

✗ **Don't** eat any snacks -
Snacks aren't included on the ACTIVE Phase

✗ **Don't** forget the ACTIVE Phase is designed to last 1-2 weeks
You can use any remaining ACTIVE Shakes on the TRIM Phase.

So what's different about the ACTIVE Shakes?

The Celebrity Slim ACTIVE Shakes are a complete meal replacement and can be consumed at any time during the Celebrity Slim Programme. The main difference is that ACTIVE Shakes are designed to be made with skimmed milk, rather than water, and are available in tubs rather than individual sachets. The shakes also include an added ingredient called L-Carnitine, which is found in many sports nutrition products.

Like all of our products the ACTIVE Shakes are based on a high protein formula, fortified with vitamins and minerals to support your energy levels.

Look out for new ACTIVE meal replacement options on our website and instore.

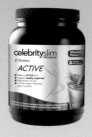
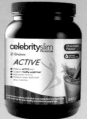

AN EXAMPLE OF A TYPICAL WEEK ON THE

	Day 1	Day 2	Day 3
Breakfast	Celebrity Slim ACTIVE Shake	Celebrity Slim ACTIVE Bar	Celebrity Slim ACTIVE Shake
Mid Morning	Celebrity Slim ACTIVE Bar	Celebrity Slim ACTIVE Shake	Celebrity Slim ACTIVE Bar
Lunch	Cheese and bacon omelette & salad	Celebrity Slim ACTIVE Shake	Celebrity Slim ACTIVE Shake
Dinner	Celebrity Slim ACTIVE Shake	Oriental Beef Stir Fry	Chicken wrappe in bacon & toma sauce with vegetab

The ACTIVE Phase is a little more restrictive in terms of food allowance than the Trim Phase as it involves having **three ACTIVE meal replacements** and **one balanced meal** per day. There are **no allowable snacks** unlike the regular TRIM Phase, which means that there is more control over your daily carbohydrate intake. Since you are exercising it is especially important to stick to the guidelines and **drink at least 2L of water** each day.

Because of the food restrictions on the ACTIVE Phase, we only recommend staying on it for short periods of 1 to 2 weeks, to help boost your weight loss. After a week or two on the ACTIVE Phase we would recommend you move to the TRIM Phase which will guide you to longer term, sustainable weight loss.

The ACTIVE Phase

ACTIVE PHASE

Day 4	Day 5	Day 6	Day 7
Celebrity Slim ACTIVE Bar	Celebrity Slim ACTIVE Shake	Celebrity Slim ACTIVE Shake	Celebrity Slim ACTIVE Bar
Celebrity Slim ACTIVE Shake	Celebrity Slim ACTIVE Bar	Celebrity Slim ACTIVE Shake	Celebrity Slim ACTIVE Shake
Celebrity Slim ACTIVE Shake	Celebrity Slim ACTIVE Shake	Celebrity Slim ACTIVE Bar	Roast chicken, carrots, cabbage & green beans
Oven baked fish ved with steamed vegetables	Grilled steak served with garden salad	Lamb chops with fennel, roast tomatoes & spinach	Celebrity Slim ACTIVE Shake

You can still use your ACTIVE Shakes on the TRIM Phase, replacing up to two of your meals per day, alongside our other meal replacement products; shakes, soups and meal bars.

You can enjoy your ACTIVE meal replacements at any time during the day but it makes sense to space out your 4 eating occasions. You can eat your meal at lunchtime or in the evening to fit in with your plans.

Don't forget - during all of the Celebrity Slim Phases, it is important to follow the allowable food and water intake guidelines as set out in the Programme Guide.

EXERCISE

One of the great things about the Celebrity Slim TRIM Phase is that your results are mainly diet dependant - that is, you don't have to do any special exercise to achieve your goals. However, the really good news is that if you do combine the Celebrity Slim TRIM Phase with regular exercise, your rate of fat loss will increase significantly and we would always encourage our members to try to incorporate exercise* into their week as part of a healthy lifestyle.

IF YOU ARE NOT USED TO DOING MUCH EXERCISE THEN START WITH SMALL STEPS AND INTRODUCE EXERCISE INTO YOUR LIFE BIT BY BIT. SIMPLE CHANGES ARE ENOUGH TO MAKE A HUGE DIFFERENCE. JUST REMEMBER TO START MODERATELY AND BUILD UP GRADUALLY.

Getting started with exercise
Choose a low-impact exercise which fits in with your lifestyle to start.

If you enjoy **swimming**, check out your local pool and start with a few lengths. Aim to build up the number of lengths, or the time you swim, each time you visit. Try water aerobics, which is a great low impact exercise and lots of fun.

Dust down your bike and go out and get some fresh air. **Cycling** is a great way of enjoying the outdoors while getting some good exercise and can be a fun way of getting the whole family out and about. Check out your local council websites for details of local cycle-tracks and routes so that you can enjoy the ride and avoid the traffic.

*Always check with your GP that the level of exercise planned is safe for you, especially if you haven't exercised for some time.

Exercise

Walking

Walking is a great form of exercise – it is flexible and completely free! Here are a few ways to incorporate walking into your daily routine; just a regular, short walk can make a real difference over a week or month.

- Walk to work rather than driving or taking the bus.
- Get off a stop early and take a brisk walk for the last 10-15 minutes.
- Before you step in the car ask yourself whether you could walk.
- Take a walk in the evening – a great way to unwind and share some quality time with family or your partner.
- Lunchtime can be a great time to squeeze in a brisk walk.

If the weather is against you then you can always consider combining a brisk walk and some indoor cycling at your **local gym** which is likely to offer both treadmills and exercise bikes along with the help and support of trained instructors.

Check out classes such as aerobics or Zumba which help to get you moving and make exercise more fun. Remember the trick is to start at a level which suits you and build from there.

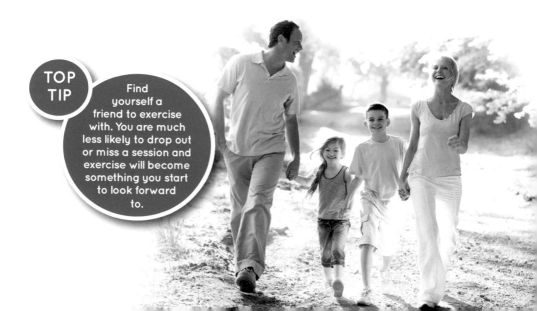

TOP TIP

Find yourself a friend to exercise with. You are much less likely to drop out or miss a session and exercise will become something you start to look forward to.

HAVING REACHED YOUR GOAL, THE MAINTAIN PHASE WILL HELP YOU TO KEEP IT OFF FOR GOOD

So you've been on the Celebrity Slim Programme for several weeks, or even months, and you've reached your goal weight. Congratulations! The Celebrity Slim MAINTAIN Phase is an essential step in keeping your weight off. During this phase we will start to reintroduce more carbohydrates into your diet.

Which carbohydrates to choose

Some carbohydrates are much healthier than others and are less likely to be converted to fat because they have a lower-GI (usually of less than 50). GI (Glyaemic Index) is a measure of how fast we digest, absorb and burn carbohydrates and it is better to choose foods which are slower to digest and so have a lower GI. As a simple rule of thumb when choosing what to eat it is often the less-processed or refined carbohydrates that are the best choices. Try to make sensible choices and eat moderate amounts of lower GI carbohydrate. If you do eat a high GI food, have a smaller portion size and perhaps combine it with a lower GI food. For example, rather than eat a big bowl of ice cream, cut back the serving size and combine it with some strawberries.

SWAP

Cornflakes or weetabix	for	natural muesli or All Bran (not Bran Flakes)
Mashed potato	for	celeriac
White rice	for	brown rice
White bread	for	wholemeal bread
Banana or pineapple	for	berries, oranges or apples
Ice-cream	for	frozen yoghurt
Peas	for	broccoli

All of the recipes you used for balanced meals during the TRIM Phase can also be used on your MAINTAIN Phase, but you can now choose to add in some low GI carbohydrate.

REINTRODUCING CARBOHYDRATE SLOWLY

It makes sense to increase your carbohydrate intake slowly as this will bring you to a stable weight and allows you to get to know what level of carbohydrate you can reintroduce into your diet without putting on weight.

Step One
- Aim to eat 2 balanced meals each day.
- Start by introducing carbohydrates into one of these meals each day, consisting of around one third of the meal portion size.
- Continue to replace 1 meal each day with a Celebrity Slim Meal Replacement product.
  We would suggest you stick to this plan for 1-2 weeks.

Step Two
- If you still continue to lose weight, increase the amount of carbohydrates by adding a portion of carbohydrate into your 2nd balanced meal.
- If you start to gain weight, cut back the carbohydrates again.

Step Three
- Replace your Celebrity Slim Programme Meal Replacement with a third meal. You can choose whether or not to add carbohydrates to this meal depending on whether this causes you to gain weight.

You may find that continuing to enjoy one carbohydrate-free meal each day helps you maintain your ideal weight.

The Maintain Phase

CHECKLIST - THE MAINTAIN PHASE

✓ **DO** eat 6 meals per day

The same schedule as on the TRIM Phase

✓ **DO** eat fewer carbs than before you started the diet

About 1/4 – 1/2 the amount of carbohydrate foods you used to eat

✓ **DO** drink 8 glasses of water per day

✓ **DO** eat lots more fruit and veg

At least 3 servings of vegetables and 2 servings of fruit per day

✗ **DON'T** skip breakfast

If you're in a hurry, have a Celebrity Slim Shake

✗ **DON'T** eat too many sugary foods

- as these are usually high GI

✗ **DON'T** forget to exercise

An essential part of a healthy lifestyle

AN EXAMPLE OF A TYPICAL WEEK ON

Many people who have successfully attained their goal weight choose to continue to use 1 Celebrity Slim Programme Meal Replacement a day, perhaps a shake for breakfast or a soup for lunch. Or they may just use Celebrity Slim Programme products for convenience on weekdays and eat normally at the weekend. This is a matter of personal choice.

	Day 1	Day 2	Day 3
Breakfast	Celebrity Slim Meal Replacement Bar	Celebrity Slim Shake	Poached egg on wholemea toast
Mid Morning	Apple	Celebrity Slim Snack Bar	Peach
Lunch	Ham salad sandwich on wholemeal bread	Salmon salad	Celebrity Slim Meal Replacem Bar
Mid Afternoon	Low fat yogurt	Orange	Vegetable stic & hummus di
Dinner	Omelette and salad	Beef & mushroom stir fry with brown rice	Chicken wrappe bacon & toma sauce & vegeta
Supper	Handful of nuts	Low fat yogurt	Fruit salad with a sma dob of crear

Step 1 (indicating the addition of 1 carbohydrate meal each day)

THE MAINTAIN PHASE

The great thing is that, if you do put on a small amount of weight, then a week or 2 on the Celebrity Slim Programme should set things right.

Day 4	Day 5	Day 6	Day 7
Celebrity Slim Shake	30g serving of cereal	Celebrity Slim Shake	Grilled bacon, mushrooms & poached egg
Orange	Vegetable sticks and dip	Celebrity Slim Snack Bar	Handful of nuts
Ham and egg salad	Celebrity Slim Soup	Egg & cress sandwich on wholemeal bread	Celebrity Slim Meal Replacement Bar
Celebrity Slim Snack Bar	Apple	Low Fat Yogurt	Vegetable sticks and dip
Chicken with holemeal pasta a cream sauce	Grilled steak with garden salad	Oven baked fish with steamed vegetables	Roast beef, vegetables & 4 new potatoes with gravy
Low fat yogurt	Handful of nuts	Fruit salad with a small dob of cream	Celery sticks and cream cheese

COMMON QUESTIONS

Is the Celebrity Slim Programme Safe?

The Celebrity Slim Programme Meal Replacements are delicious high protein foods. They are formulated using a blend of common food ingredients and are perfectly safe for use by normal healthy adults.

Is Celebrity Slim suitable for men and women?

Men are absolutely fine to follow the programme. They may find that they are a little hungrier during week 1, in which case we would just suggest adding 1 more healthy snack for that week. Opt for more protein based snacks during week 1 also – ham, nuts, cheese, Celebrity Slim snack bars etc. The protein serving for the balanced meal is slightly larger for a man so 100 – 200g (roughly the size and thickness of the palm of your hand).

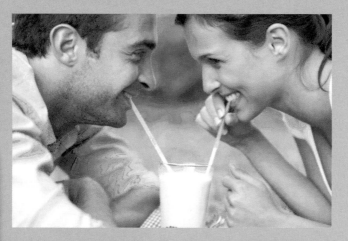

Is the Programme safe for children?

The Celebrity Slim Programme is classified as a formulated dietary food and is designed to be used by people over 16 years of age.

- ## Can I follow the Celebrity Slim Programme if I'm pregnant or breastfeeding?

  Because the Celebrity Slim Programme is based on a reduced Calorie diet, we do not recommend it for women who are pregnant or breastfeeding as the diet may not contain enough nutrients to support the needs of both mum and baby.

- ## Can I follow the Celebrity Slim Programme if I am lactose intolerant?

  One of the ingredients in the Celebrity Slim Programme shakes, soups and bars is 'skimmed milk powder' which does contain lactose, so the shakes are not suitable if you are lactose intolerant.

- ## Can I follow the Celebrity Slim Programme if I have Coeliac Disease?

  Some of the flavours used in the Celebrity Slim Programme may contain traces of gluten so if you have this condition the Celebrity Slim Programme would not be suitable.

- ## Can I replace all of my meals with the Celebrity Slim Meal Replacements?

  Some people use meal replacement shakes as their only food to lose weight quickly. While this may work in the short term it is not a balanced way to eat for any longer than a few days. We always recommend combining the Celebrity Slim Programme shakes with healthy balanced meals and snacks to ensure you are getting a good intake of fresh food nutrients every day to help you control your weight and stay healthy.

- ## How long will it take to reach my target weight?

  Naturally, individual weight loss will vary. Some people may lose weight faster than others, particularly if they combine the programme with some regular exercise. If you are diligently following the programme and not seeing much short term change, hang in there. Your body may need a little time to stabilise and get used to this new way of eating. Usually after about a week or so, your body and metabolism adapt, and you will start losing weight and feeling great.

• What if I'm still hungry?

If you're sticking to the quantities suggested on the Celebrity Slim Programme and still seem to be hungry, there are a few strategies you can use. First of all, make sure you are truly hungry and not just wanting to eat out of habit or through thirst. Secondly, bear in mind that in the first week you may feel hungry as you are adjusting to a new way of eating.

• Things you can do to beat hunger

- Drink more water with your meals and snacks.
- Increase the portion size of each meal and snack by about 10% for a few days, and then slowly reduce it if you can.
- Add a small handful of allowed nuts with a glass of water to one snack.
- Keep slices of vegetables, such as celery, carrot and peppers in the fridge to munch on when needed.

• If I get constipated what should I do?

If this happens to you, check you are drinking at least 2 litres of water and eating plenty of fresh vegetables and fruit as these are a good source of fibre. Sometimes a change in eating habits can cause irregularity so make sure you follow the guidelines. If symptoms persist then you should visit your Pharmacist for advice, or contact our customer services by phone or email. See page 37 for contact information.

•Why has my weight loss plateaued?

Your body has many systems and processes built in to adapt to and counter changing conditions and it may be that your body is simply fighting your attempts to lose weight by slowing your Metabolic Rate.

A few tips to kick start your weight loss again:
- Try substituting a fruit snack with a protein rich snack like a boiled egg or lean meat. Do this for 4 or 5 days.
- Add exercise to your routine.
- If you already exercise – vary what you do to force your body to work harder.

- Swap your meals, maybe have your balanced meal at lunchtime and make sure you have snacks in between meals.
- Drink plenty of water - you need at least 2 litres per day in small, regular quantities.
- Ensure you have adequate fibre intake through your vegetable servings.
- If you feel you don't need your snacks skip them for a few days.

Alternatively try the ACTIVE Phase for 1 to 2 weeks to give your weight loss a kick-start. This phase can help to accelerate your weight loss goals. Find out more at celebrityslim.co.uk or in the ACTIVE Phase section of this guide.

• If I stop using the Celebrity Slim Programme, will I put on weight?

There's no reason why you will put on weight if you stop using the Celebrity Slim Programme as long as you maintain a sensible approach to your diet. Follow the Celebrity Slim Programme **MAINTAIN Phase** outlined in this booklet and you should be able to keep to the weight level you have achieved.

• What should I do if I start putting on weight while I'm on the MAINTAIN Phase?

If you find weight is creeping back on, perhaps because you've been a little relaxed with your eating, simply go back on the Celebrity Slim **TRIM Phase** until you are happy with your weight.

For more FAQs about the Celebrity Slim Programme go to our website at celebrityslim.co.uk

Recipe Ideas

TOP TIP

Experiment with herbs and spices to add flavour but not Calories to your dishes

SIMPLE MEAL IDEAS

Serve all of these recipes with good helpings of allowable vegetables or salad to meet the balanced meal guidelines of the Celebrity Slim Programme. All recipes serve 2 unless otherwise stated

Chicken with Mustard

Make a few cuts in 2 chicken breasts. Mix 2 tbsp wholegrain mustard with one tbsp of olive oil and spread over the top. Grill for 20-25 minutes or until cooked through.

Salmon with Ginger, Chilli & Garlic

Place 2 salmon steaks or fillets on a large square of foil. Top with 2 tsp grated ginger, 1 finely chopped red chilli, a thin sliced clove of garlic and 1 tbsp chopped coriander. Seal the foil like a loose parcel and bake for 25 mins at 180°C.

Chicken with Lemon & Garlic

Mix the juice from 1 lemon, 1 tbsp olive oil, and 1 crushed garlic clove and use to marinate 2 chicken breasts for 20 minutes. Remove from marinade and grill for 20-25 minutes or fry gently in a little olive oil until cooked through. Sprinkle with chopped parsley.

Oriental Salmon (Pictured opposite)

Mix 2 tbsp soy sauce with 1 tbsp oyster sauce and use to marinade 2 salmon steaks or fillets for 20 mins. Fry or grill.

Chicken & Chorizo Kebabs

Mix 1tbsp olive oil, 1tsp dried oregano, ½ tsp paprika and use to marinate 2 small chicken breasts for 20 minutes. Slice a 3-inch chorizo sausage into 1cm slices. Cut the chicken into bite-size chunks and thread the chicken, chorizo and chunks of green or red pepper onto 2 skewers and grill for 20-25 minutes.

Broccoli & Parmesan Frittata

Beat 4 eggs and mix in 1 tbsp grated parmesan, salt and pepper.
Boil broccoli for 3-4 minutes. Fry ½ small onion chopped, until soft.
Add the broccoli and egg mixture to the pan. Cook slowly over a low
heat for 15 minutes until almost set. Pop under a grill to set the top.

Cheese & Garlic Mushroom Omelette

Fry a large handful of mixed sliced mushrooms in ½ tbsp olive oil with
1 crushed clove of garlic until soft. Beat 2 eggs with salt and pepper
and add to a hot omelette pan. Just before the omelette sets sprinkle
with 1 tbsp grated cheese, fill with the mushrooms and serve (serves 1).

Lamb, Mint & Yogurt Patties (Pictured below)

In a food processor, process ½ lb of lamb mince with 1 chopped
onion, 1 clove of garlic, 1 tbsp of chopped mint, salt and pepper.
Form into 4 patties. Grill for 15 mins and serve with a side dish of plain
yogurt mixed with chopped cucumber and mint.

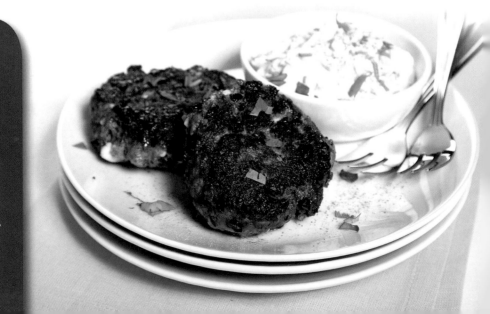

Chicken Tikka Skewers Serves 4

What you'll need

- 15g low fat yogurt
- 2 tbsp hot curry paste
- 4 boneless skinless chicken breasts, cubed
- 250g cherry tomatoes
- ½ cucumber, cubed
- 1 red onion, thinly sliced
- juice of 1 lemon
- 50g salad leaves

The easy bit

1. Place 8 wooden skewers in a bowl of cold water to soak.
2. Mix together the yogurt and curry paste in a bowl add cubed chicken and to marinate for one hour.
3. Toss cucumber, onion and lemon juice in large bowl and chill in fridge.
4. Remove chicken from marinade and thread onto skewers with the cherry tomatoes.
5. Cook under a medium grill for 15-20 minutes until cooked through and golden.
6. Stir salad leaves into the chilled dressing and divide between 4 plates and top with 2 skewers each.

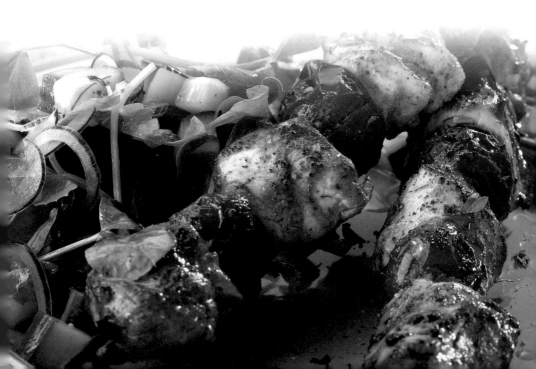

Rosemary Lamb Cutlets with Roasted Fennel & Spinach

What you'll need

- 6 lamb cutlets
- 2 tablespoons olive oil
- 1 tbsp chopped fresh rosemary
- 1 tbsp finely grated lemon zest
- salt and black pepper
- 1 medium fennel bulb, cut into thick slices
- 6-8 cloves garlic, unpeeled
- 100 g baby spinach

The easy bit

1. Place lamb cutlets in a shallow dish, add 1 tablespoon oil, the rosemary, lemon zest, salt and pepper and mix well.
2. Refrigerate for 2-3 hours.
3. Preheat oven to 190°C.
4. In a roasting dish, place the fennel and garlic, then drizzle over the remaining oil and season with salt and pepper.
5. Roast for 20 minutes.
6. Meanwhile, heat a grill plate or frying pan until smoking, then add the lamb and cook for approximately 4 minutes on each side.
7. Remove the fennel and garlic from the oven, squeeze the garlic cloves from their skins and discard the skins.
8. Stir through the spinach leaves - the heat from the fennel will wilt the spinach a little - and serve with the lamb cutlets.

Tip: This is a great recipe to cook on the barbecue in summer.

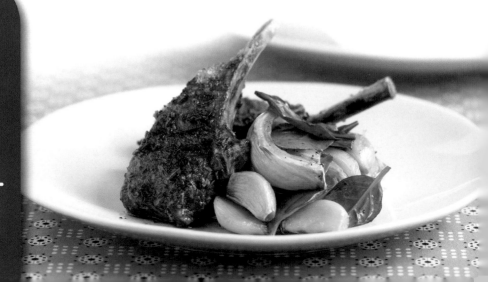

Chargrilled Sirloin Steak with Horseradish Cream & Celeriac Mash

What you'll need

- 2 sirloin steaks, about 180g each
- 1 tablespoon olive oil
- salt and black pepper
- 200g celeriac bulb, peeled and cut into chunks
- 1 teaspoon horseradish
- 2 tbsps light sour cream
- 2 tsps chopped fresh chives

The easy bit

1. Season the steaks with the oil, salt and pepper and set aside.
2. Place the celeriac in a saucepan and cover with water, bring to a boil and cook until tender, about 10 minutes.
3. Meanwhile, mix together the horseradish, sour cream and chives and set aside.
4. Preheat oven to 180°C.
5. Heat a grill plate or frying pan until smoking hot, add the steak and seal the meat on both sides - this will help keep in the juices.
6. Transfer to the oven and cook until done to your liking.
7. Drain the celeriac and lightly mash with a fork. Season to taste with salt and pepper.
8. Place the mash on a plate, then top with the steak and a dollop of horseradish cream.
9. Serve with a green side salad.

TOP TIP
If celeriac is not available you can use cauliflower instead. Cauliflower mash makes a great healthy alternative to mashed potatoes

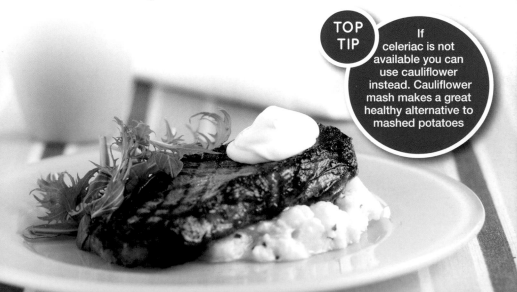

Steamed Salmon with Ginger, Chilli and Garlic

What you'll need

- 2 salmon fillets, 120g each
- 1 teaspoon sesame oil
- ½ red chilli, deseeded and sliced
- 2 teaspoons grated fresh ginger
- 2 cloves garlic, sliced
- 1 lime, sliced
- 1 tbsp chopped fresh coriander, plus extra for garnish
- salt and black pepper
- 1 bunch pak choi
- 1 spring onion, sliced

The easy bit

1. Cut 2 pieces of greaseproof paper each large enough to wrap a piece of salmon.
2. Place a piece of salmon onto each piece of paper.
3. Top each piece of fish with sesame oil, chilli, ginger, garlic, lime and coriander and season with salt and pepper.
4. Fold the paper over the salmon and fold up at the ends to make a tight parcel so none of the juices can escape.
5. Place in a steamer and steam for 10 minutes until cooked.
6. Remove fish from the steamer, set aside.
7. Add the pak choi and steam for 4-5 minutes, remove fish from parcel.
8. Place the salmon onto plates, and sprinkle over the spring onion.
9. Garnish with extra coriander and serve with the steamed pak choi.

Tip: To try something a little different, you can substitute the salmon for fresh tuna.

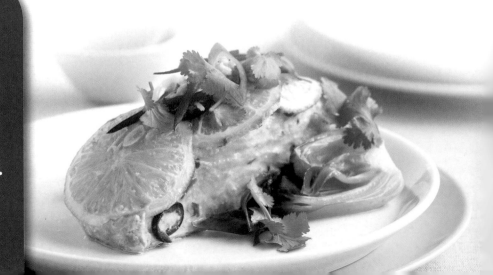

The great thing about the Celebrity Slim Programme is that you get to enjoy a delicious meal each day, and if you're looking for ideas and inspiration - look no further than the Celebrity Slim website.

Whether you are planning a quick family supper or a special occasion there will be something to suit. To access the full list of recipes you simply need to join the Celebrity Slim Club online. Joining is quick, easy, completely confidential and FREE!

Here are just some of the delicious recipes you'll find:

PORK, LAMB or BEEF
Grilled lemon pork cutlet with warm red cabbage.
Lamb with chilli tomato salsa.
Sticky pork with asian greens.
Pork and pepper stir fry.
Cauliflower topped cottage pie.
Steak with pea puree, mushrooms and asparagus.
Hearty lamb hotpot with cauliflower mash.
Crispy bacon and egg benedict.

CHICKEN
Stir Fried chicken with chilli and coriander.
BBQ peri peri chicken breast with asparagus, fennel & orange salad.
Roast chicken with lemon glaze.
Ricotta stuffed chicken with prosciutto.

VEGETARIAN
Cajun Mushrooms.
Malaysian mushroom omelette.
Aubergine and ricotta rolls.
Halloumi and asparagus salad.
Cauliflower cheese.
Vegetarian Sicilian stew.

SEAFOOD
Tuna kebabs with indian salad.
Chorizo & prawn skewers.
Steamed mussels with coconut milk.
Roast cod with sweet & sour peppers & salsa verde.
Mediterranean fish bake.

SOUPS
Roast tomato & basil soup.
French onion soup with parmesan.
Hearty vegetable soup

For more fantastic recipe ideas visit celebrityslim.co.uk/recipes

Recipe Lists

CELEBRITY SLIM PRODUCTS

Meal replacements

All of our meal replacements are designed to taste delicious whilst offering all of the essential nutrients you should expect from a meal.

Shakes

Available in a range of delicious flavours such as Strawberry, Vanilla, Cafe Latte, Banana and Chocolate.

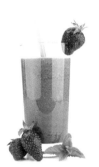
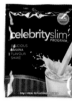
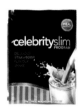
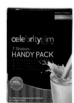
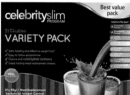

Active Shakes

Available in chocolate or strawberry ACTIVE shakes contain the sports supplement L-Carnitine. They should be made with milk and can be used during any phase of the programme.

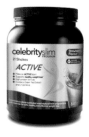
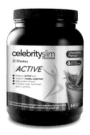

Soups

Perfect for lunch when you feel like a hot meal, our soups provide a tasty, savoury alternative in a range of flavours including Roast Chicken, Garden Vegetable and Mild Curry (Mulligatawny).

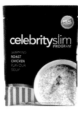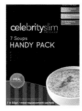

Meal Replacement Bars

These delicious bars offer a satisfying meal option in delicious flavours such as Fruit and Nut or Chocolate Caramel. Great for when you are out and about.

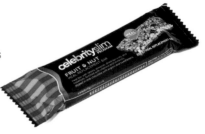

Snacks

These handy bars are great to keep in your handbag for your snacking moments. Available in great flavours such as Rocky Road and Sticky Toffee.

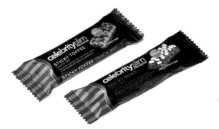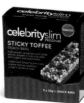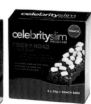

Use these lists as an easy reference guide to help you make better food choices

✓ PROTEIN FOODS TO ENJOY

Enjoy a portion of protein with every balanced meal – it should be around the size and thickness of the palm of your hand.

LEAN MEAT & POULTRY

Remove excess fat before cooking and choose lean cuts e.g. pork chops, lamb steaks, lean or low-fat mince. Remove any skin from poultry.

Beef	Lean Cooked Ham	Turkey
Chicken	Lean Cooked Turkey	Veal
Lamb	Pork	

FISH & SEAFOOD

Any fish fillets or seafood. For example:

Cod	Mussels	Sea Bass
Haddock	Prawns	Trout
Lobster	Salmon	Tuna
Mackerel	Sardines	

OTHER PROTEIN SOURCES

Choose low-fat options

Cottage Cheese	Halloumi	Ricotta
Feta Cheese	Quorn	Tofu

Cheddar and Parmesan – use in moderation to flavour dishes

ADDING FLAVOUR TO MEALS

Balsamic vinegar	Lemon juice	Spices
Garlic	Low-fat dressings	Tomato puree
Herbs	Soy sauce	

✗ CARBOHYDRATES TO AVOID

Bread	Pasta	Potatoes
Couscous	Pizza	Rice

✓ VEGETABLES TO ENJOY

Artichoke	Celeriac	Olives
Asparagus	Celery	Onions
Aubergine	Courgettes	Pak Choi
Basil	Cucumber	Parsley
Beetroot	Fennel	Peppers
Brussel sprouts	Garlic	Pickles
Broccoli	Lettuce	Radish
Capers	Leeks	Spinach
Cabbage	Mange Tout	Spring Onions
Cauliflower	Mushrooms	Tomatoes

✓ VEGETABLES TO ENJOY IN MODERATION

Avocado	Carrots	Swede
Beetroot	Green Beans	Turnip

✗ VEGETABLES TO AVOID

BECAUSE THEY ARE HIGH IN CARBOHYDRATE		Peas
Barley	Chickpeas	Potato
Beans (baked/kidney)	Lentils	Sweet Potato
Butternut Squash	Parsnips	Sweetcorn

✓ FRUIT TO ENJOY AS SNACKS

Choose ½ - ¾ cup of berries or a small whole fruit

Apple	1/2 Grapefruit	Plum
Blackberries	Orange	Raspberries
Blueberries	Peach	Strawberries
Cherries	Pear	

✗ FRUITS TO AVOID

BECAUSE THEY ARE HIGH IN CARBOHYDRATE		Mango
Apricot	Grapes	Melon (all types)
Banana	Kiwi	Pineapple

Avoid all dried fruits along with fruit tinned in syrup/nectar

✓ OTHER FOODS TO ENJOY AS SNACKS

30 grams (small block or slice) of cheese.

1-2 slices of lean deli meats such as ham (avoid salami or similar).

About 30g (small handful) of nuts - raw almonds, peanuts, Brazil nuts, walnuts or pistachio (go easy on salted nuts and avoid any coated nuts).

A tablespoon of low fat natural yogurt with fruit such as berries.

Carrot and/or celery sticks with cream cheese or a low fat dip

Smoked salmon slice spread thinly with cream cheese.

Cheese slice and a pickle wrapped in a slice of ham.

4 olives with cheese and ham.

Small tin tuna in water with lettuce, spring onion and low-fat mayo

Slice of smoked salmon spread thinly with cream cheese

Grilled mushrooms topped with cheese and herbs

Low-fat yogurt (plain or flavoured)

Hard boiled egg

✓ DRINKS TO ENJOY

Water – at least 2 litres per day

Tea or coffee, with or without milk, max 3 cups per day - use artificial sweetener and avoid lattes or cappucino

Diet soft drinks and diet cordials - maximum 2 glasses per day

Dry white or red wine* - maximum 3 glasses per week

Spirit with a diet mixer* – maximum 3 glasses per week

Low carbohydrate beer* - maximum 3 glasses per week

✗ DRINKS TO AVOID

Alcohol in excess of the amounts given above*

Cordial (full sugar)

Fruit juices

Milk – skim, low fat, full cream and flavoured all are high in carbs. but a splash of skimmed milk can be added to tea or coffee.

Fruit Smoothies

Soft drinks (full sugar)

Sports drink

*All alcohol should be avoided during the ACTIVE Phase.

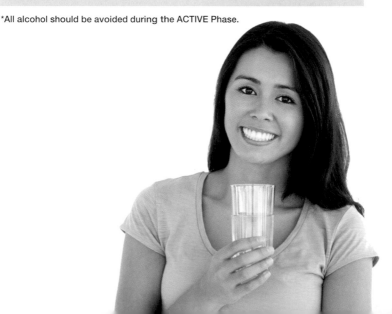

THE CELEBRITY SLIM PROGRAMME IS DESIGNED TO BE SIMPLE AND EASY TO FOLLOW SO YOU DON'T NEED TO TRACK EVERY MEAL YOU CONSUME TO STAY ON TARGET.

However, it can be helpful to keep a record of your experience of the programme, particularly when you first start.

The 'My Celebrity Slim' section is designed to give you a quick and easy way to check that you are eating regularly, drinking enough water and incorporating some physical activity into your week. We have included a space on each page where you can jot down anything which you feel will help you in the coming weeks; a favourite shake flavour, a recipe you tried and enjoyed, or just a positive thought which motivated you.

As you progress towards your goal, if you have a difficult week, you can look back to previous weeks and see what helped you then. Keeping a track of how well you follow the programme is an essential step to understanding the link between what you do and the results you achieve.

Don't forget to make them realistic – it is better to start with an achievable goal and then review your goal when you get there! Your goal might be a weight loss goal or you may want to drop a dress size or lose inches. Decide when you will weigh yourself each week and take a few measurements so that you can see how your body changes as you progress through the diet. Complete the personal record on page 78 and then start tracking your progress overleaf or download our free APP from the Celebrity Slim website.

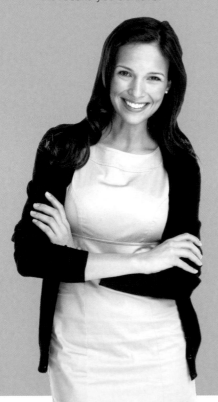
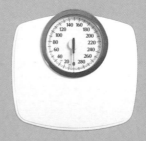

MY CELEBRITY SLIM - **WEEK 1**

	Monday	Tuesday	Wednesday	Thursday	Friday	Saturday	Sunday
Breakfast							
Snack							
Lunch							
Snack							
Dinner							
Snack							
Water							
Exercise							

STARTING WEIGHT... END OF WEEK WEIGHT...

THIS WEEK I LOST .... SO FAR I HAVE LOST...

NOTES...

....

MY CELEBRITY SLIM - **WEEK 2**

Monday	Tuesday	Wednesday	Thursday	Friday	Saturday	Sunday

STARTING WEIGHT.. END OF WEEK WEIGHT..

THIS WEEK I LOST.. SO FAR I HAVE LOST..

NOTES..

MY CELEBRITY SLIM - **WEEK 3**

	Monday	Tuesday	Wednesday	Thursday	Friday	Saturday	Sunday
Breakfast							
Snack							
Lunch							
Snack							
Dinner							
Snack							
Water							
Exercise							

STARTING WEIGHT _____ END OF WEEK WEIGHT _____

THIS WEEK I LOST _____ SO FAR I HAVE LOST _____

NOTES _____